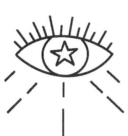

This Book Belongs To

*I recommend using pencil, colored pencil
or gel pens to reduce bleed through when
coloring in this book.

*This book is designed to keep track of your period and
your PMS symptoms for one year
as well as provide pages for reflection,
journaling and mood tracking.

*Your period is a normal, natural and
healthy occurrence.
*If you track your period every month, you
may notice a pattern. It may become easier
to tell when you will get your next period and
you may discover things that help alleviate
any discomforts
*A menstrual cycle is counted from the first day of bleeding
in one month to the first day of bleeding in the next month.
*The average menstrual cycle is about 28 days, but cycles
that are 21-45 days are also normal. It may take 6 years or
more for your cycle to become regular.

Please enjoy this book and provide any reviews and
feedback so that I can create the best journals and
trackers for you, my amazing customers!

SOME COMMON TYPES OF PERIOD PRODUCTS

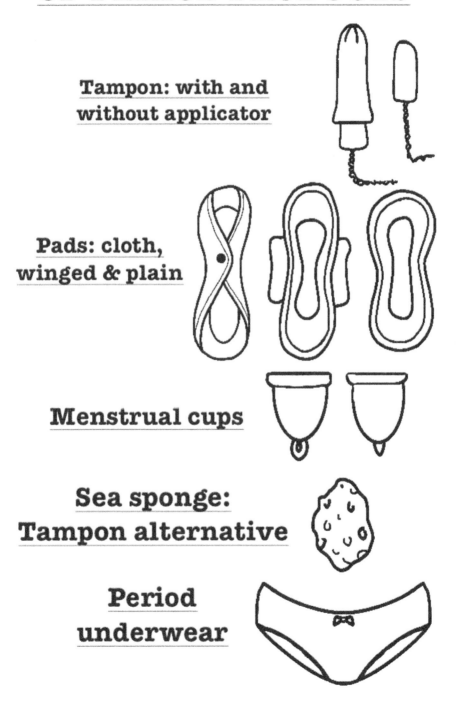

Tampon: with and without applicator

Pads: cloth, winged & plain

Menstrual cups

Sea sponge: Tampon alternative

Period underwear

Female Reproductive System

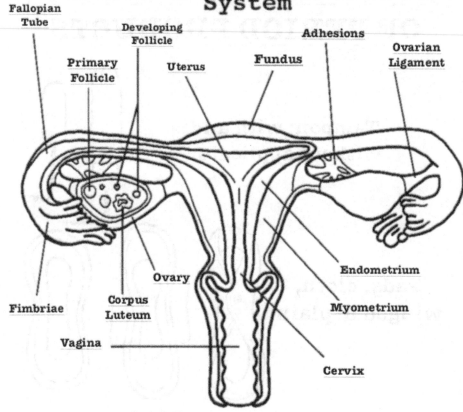

Fallopian Tube

Developing Follicle

Primary Follicle

Uterus

Fundus

Adhesions

Ovarian Ligament

Ovary

Endometrium

Fimbriae

Corpus Luteum

Myometrium

Vagina

Cervix

The Vulva

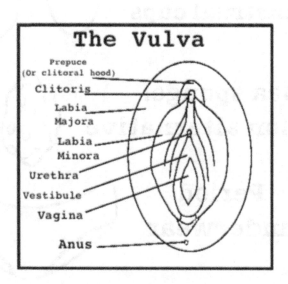

Prepuce (Or clitoral hood)

Clitoris

Labia Majora

Labia Minora

Urethra

Vestibule

Vagina

Anus

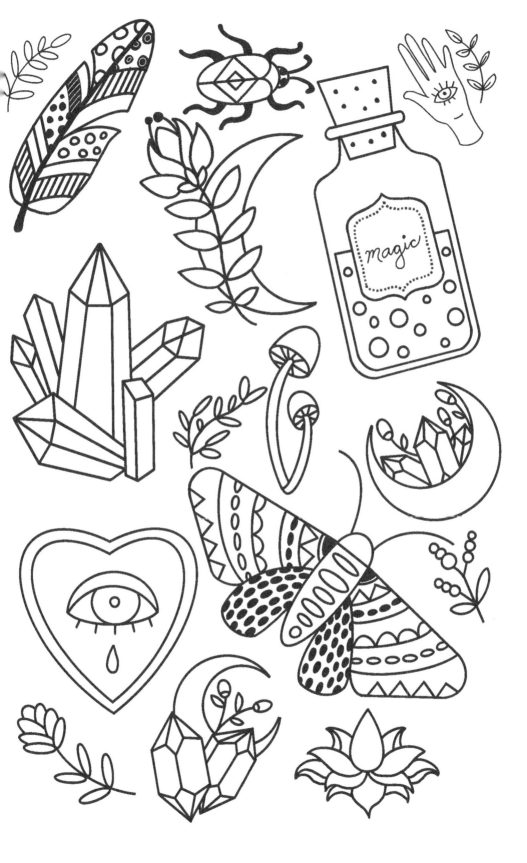

Month: _____   **Year:** _____

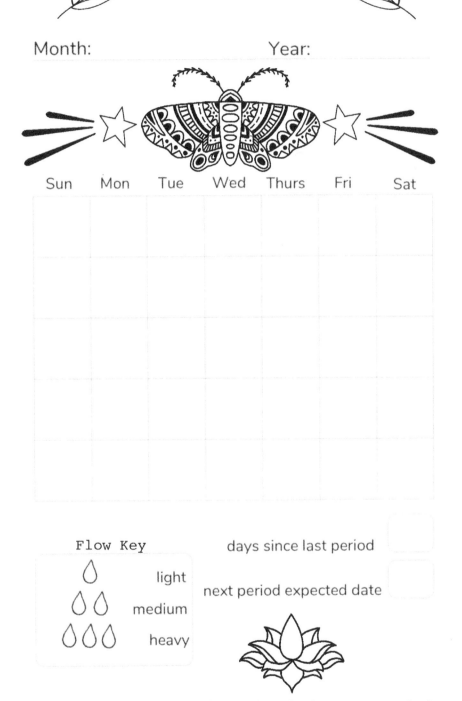

Sun	Mon	Tue	Wed	Thurs	Fri	Sat

Flow Key

⋀   light

⋀⋀   medium

⋀⋀⋀   heavy

days since last period _____

next period expected date _____

Mark the days you have your period on the calendar. You can mark them using the flow key or draw hearts, stars or anything you like.

PMS symptoms

Write down anything you may be experiencing during your period. Include your moods, any cravings, aches, cramps or tenderness you are feeling and anything you did that helped.

Day 1	
Day 2	
Day 3	
Day 4	
Day 5	
Day 6	
Day 7	

Notes:

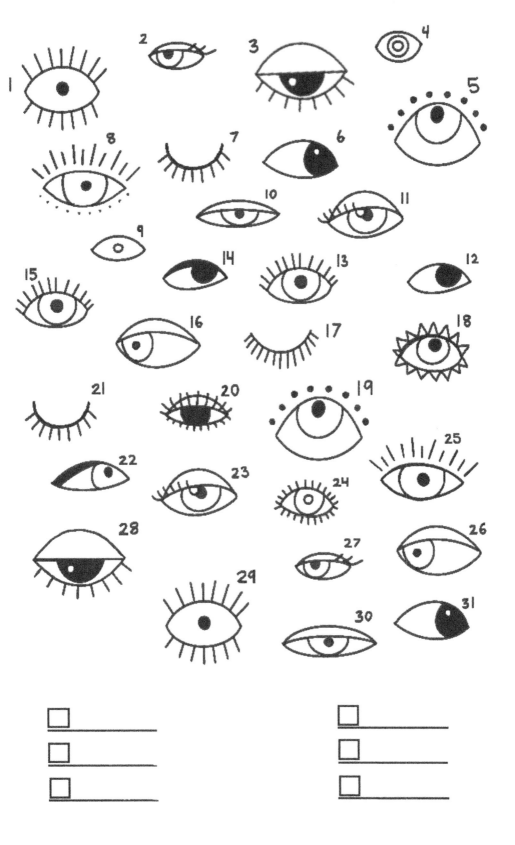

Month: Year:

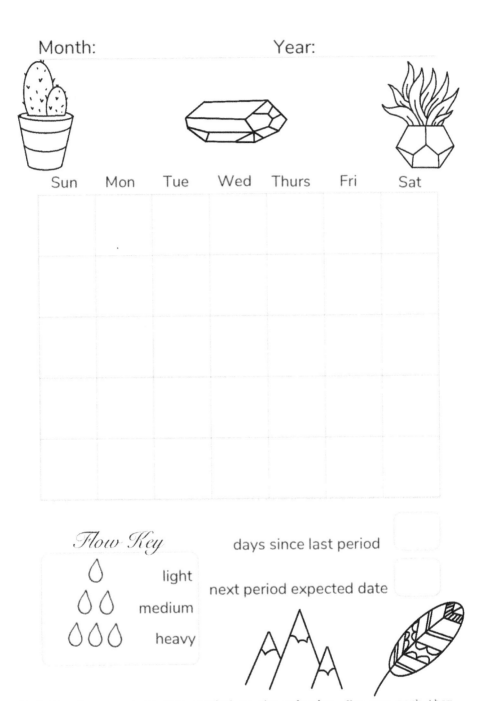

Sun	Mon	Tue	Wed	Thurs	Fri	Sat

Flow Key

💧 light

💧💧 medium

💧💧💧 heavy

days since last period

next period expected date

Mark the days you have your period on the calendar. You can mark them using the flow key or draw hearts, stars or anything you like.

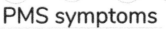

PMS symptoms

Write down anything you may be experiencing during your period. Include your moods, any cravings, aches, cramps or tenderness you are feeling and anything you did that helped.

Day 1	
Day 2	
Day 3	
Day 4	
Day 5	
Day 6	
Day 7	

Notes:

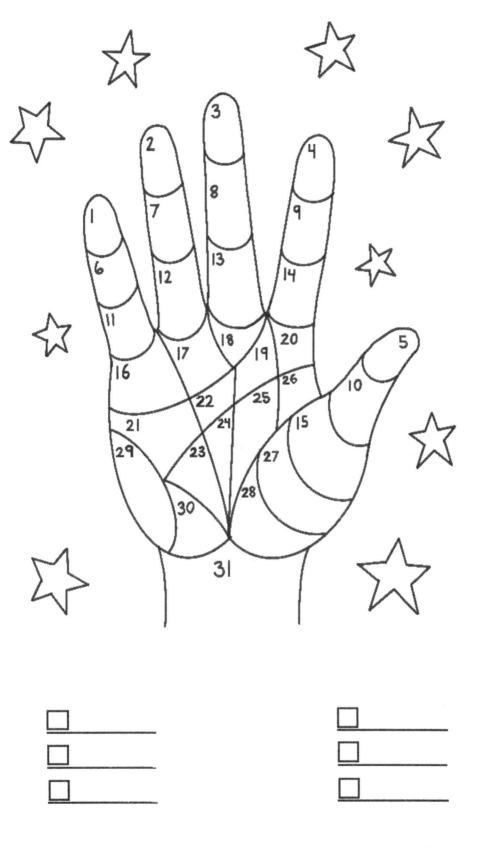

Month: _____   Year: _____

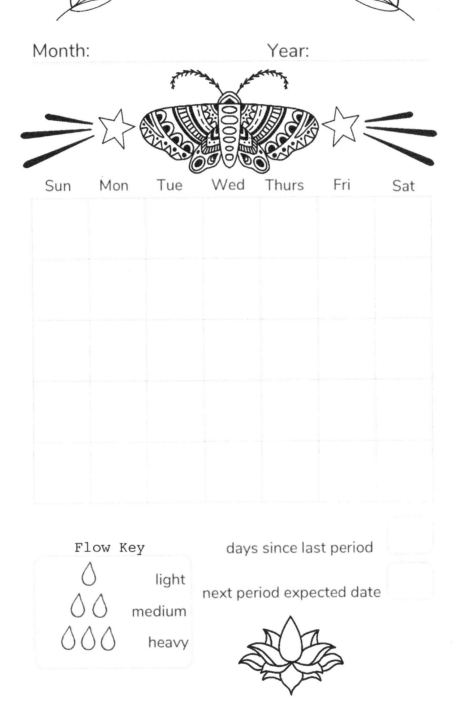

Sun	Mon	Tue	Wed	Thurs	Fri	Sat

Flow Key

light

medium

heavy

days since last period

next period expected date

Mark the days you have your period on the calendar. You can mark them using the flow key or draw hearts, stars or anything you like.

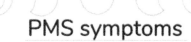

PMS symptoms

Write down anything you may be experiencing during your period. Include your moods, any cravings, aches, cramps or tenderness you are feeling and anything you did that helped.

Day 1	
Day 2	
Day 3	
Day 4	
Day 5	
Day 6	
Day 7	

Notes:

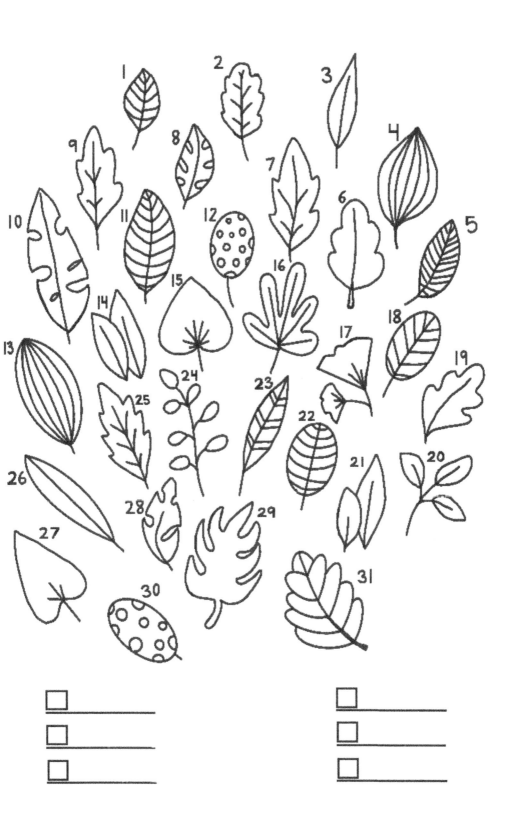

Month: _____   Year: _____

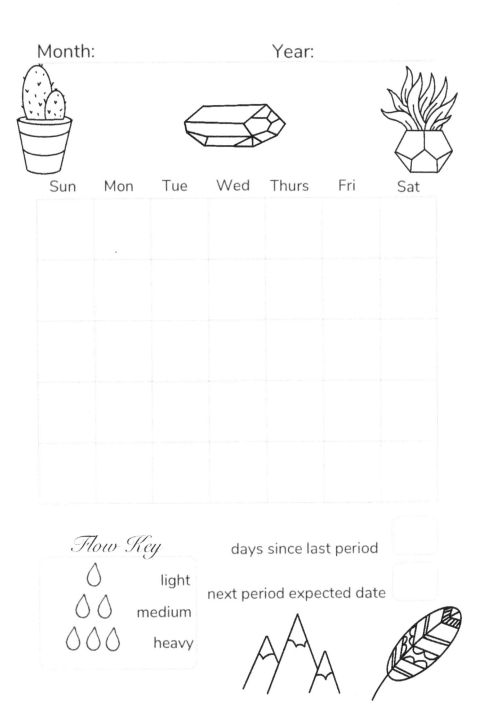

Sun	Mon	Tue	Wed	Thurs	Fri	Sat

Flow Key

light

medium

heavy

days since last period

next period expected date

Mark the days you have your period on the calendar. You can mark them using the flow key or draw hearts, stars or anything you like.

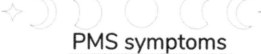

PMS symptoms

Write down anything you may be experiencing during your period. Include your moods, any cravings, aches, cramps or tenderness you are feeling and anything you did that helped.

Day 1	
Day 2	
Day 3	
Day 4	
Day 5	
Day 6	
Day 7	

Notes:

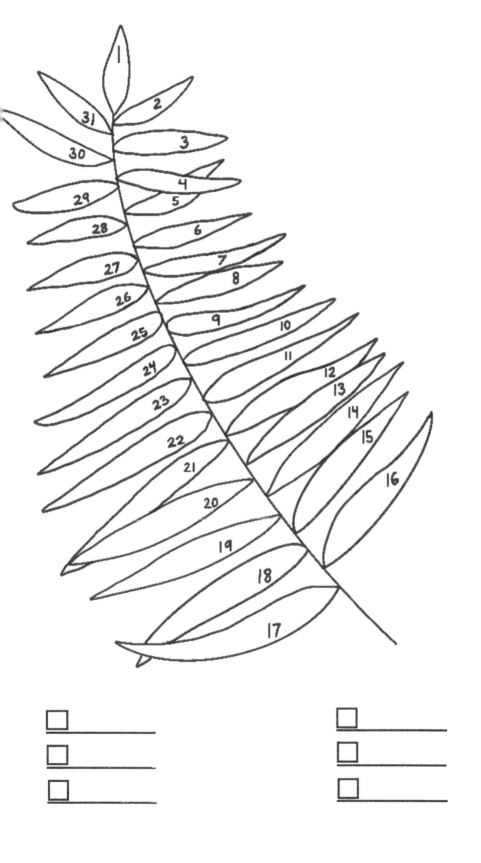

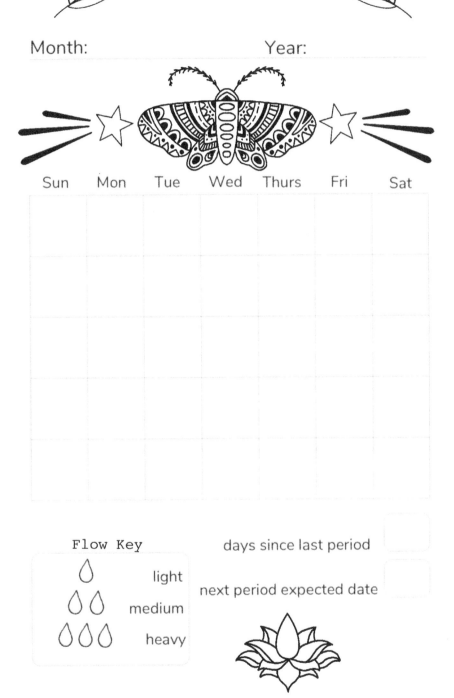

Month: _____   Year: _____

Sun	Mon	Tue	Wed	Thurs	Fri	Sat

Flow Key

○ light

○○ medium

○○○ heavy

days since last period

next period expected date

Mark the days you have your period on the calendar. You can mark them using the flow key or draw hearts, stars or anything you like.

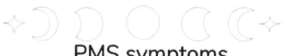

PMS symptoms

Write down anything you may be experiencing during your period. Include your moods, any cravings, aches, cramps or tenderness you are feeling and anything you did that helped.

Day 1	
Day 2	
Day 3	
Day 4	
Day 5	
Day 6	
Day 7	

Notes:

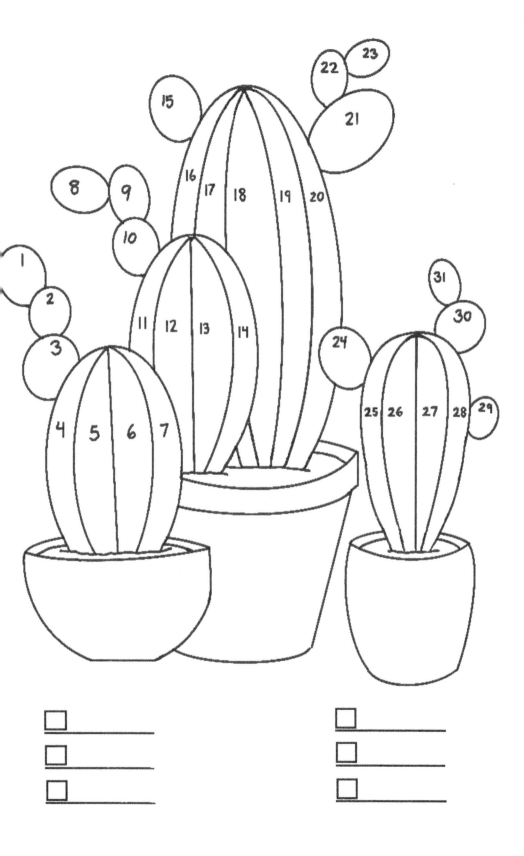

Month: Year:

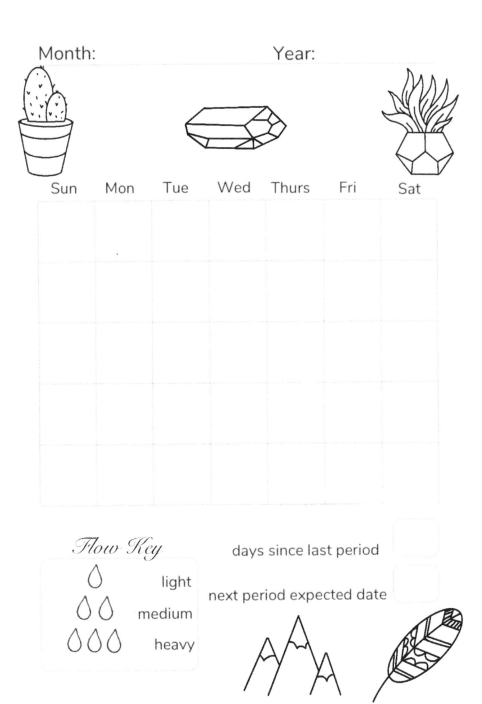

Sun	Mon	Tue	Wed	Thurs	Fri	Sat

Flow Key

◊ light

◊ ◊ medium

◊ ◊ ◊ heavy

days since last period

next period expected date

Mark the days you have your period on the calendar. You can mark them
using the flow key or draw hearts, stars or anything you like.

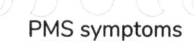

PMS symptoms

Write down anything you may be experiencing during your period. Include your moods, any cravings, aches, cramps or tenderness you are feeling and anything you did that helped.

Day 1	
Day 2	
Day 3	
Day 4	
Day 5	
Day 6	
Day 7	

Notes:

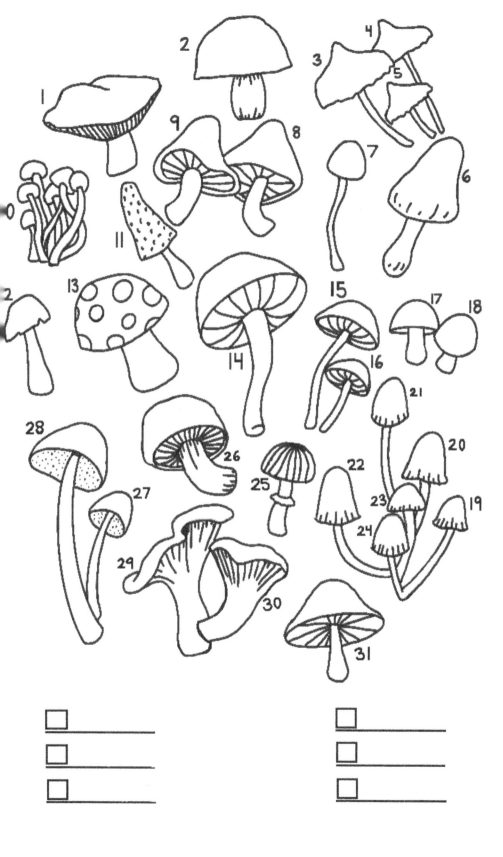

Month: _____ Year: _____

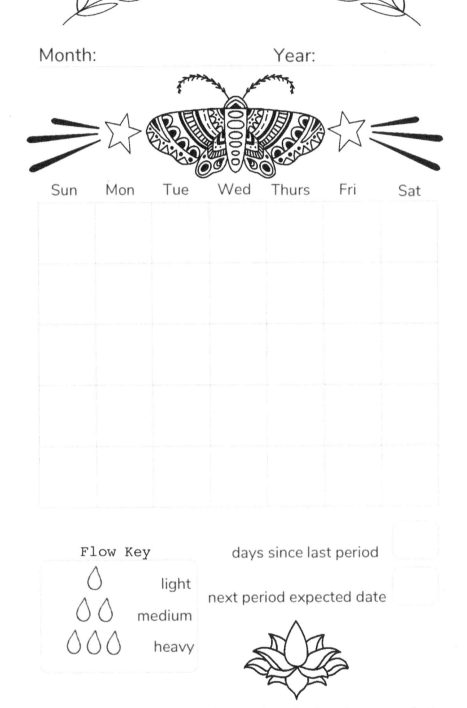

Sun	Mon	Tue	Wed	Thurs	Fri	Sat

Flow Key

⬠ light

⬠⬠ medium

⬠⬠⬠ heavy

days since last period

next period expected date

Mark the days you have your period on the calendar. You can mark them using the flow key or draw hearts, stars or anything you like.

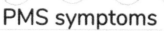

PMS symptoms

Write down anything you may be experiencing during your period. Include your moods, any cravings, aches, cramps or tenderness you are feeling and anything you did that helped.

Day 1	
Day 2	
Day 3	
Day 4	
Day 5	
Day 6	
Day 7	

Notes:

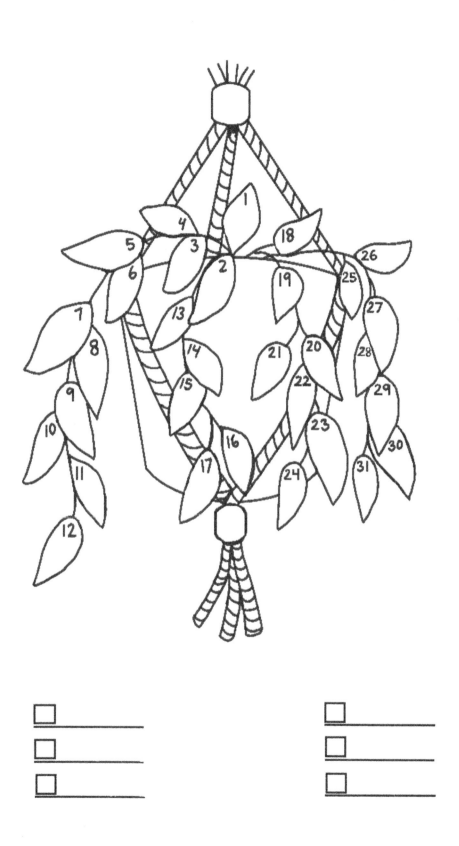

Month: _____   Year: _____

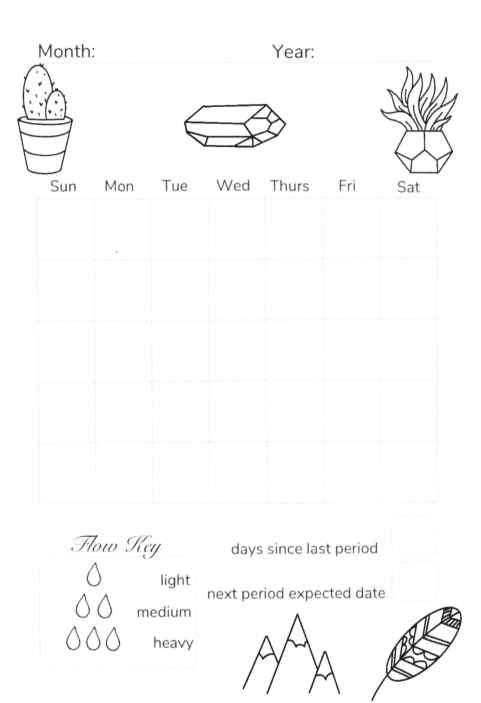

	Sun	Mon	Tue	Wed	Thurs	Fri	Sat

Flow Key

◊ light
◊◊ medium
◊◊◊ heavy

_____ days since last period

_____ next period expected date

Mark the days you have your period on the calendar. You can mark them
using the flow key or draw hearts, stars or anything you like.

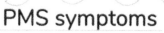

PMS symptoms

Write down anything you may be experiencing during your period. Include your moods, any cravings, aches, cramps or tenderness you are feeling and anything you did that helped.

Day 1	
Day 2	
Day 3	
Day 4	
Day 5	
Day 6	
Day 7	

Notes:

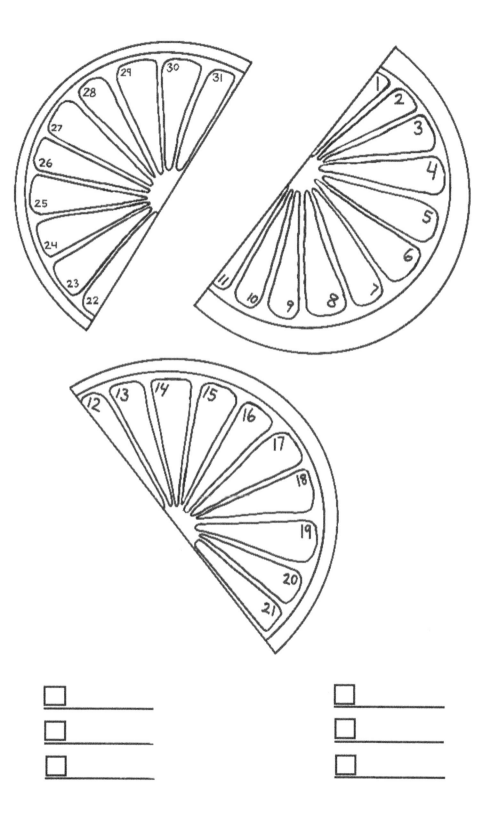

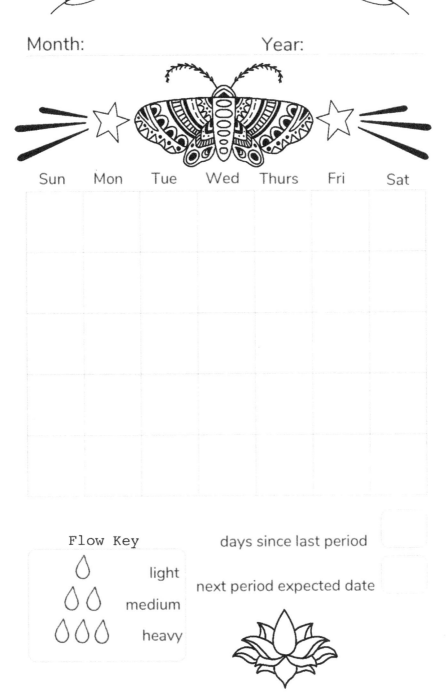

Month: _____   Year: _____

Sun	Mon	Tue	Wed	Thurs	Fri	Sat

Flow Key

◊ light

◊◊ medium

◊◊◊ heavy

days since last period ☐

next period expected date ☐

Mark the days you have your period on the calendar. You can mark them using the flow key or draw hearts, stars or anything you like.

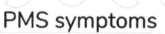

PMS symptoms

Write down anything you may be experiencing during your period. Include your moods, any cravings, aches, cramps or tenderness you are feeling and anything you did that helped.

Day 1	
Day 2	
Day 3	
Day 4	
Day 5	
Day 6	
Day 7	

Notes:

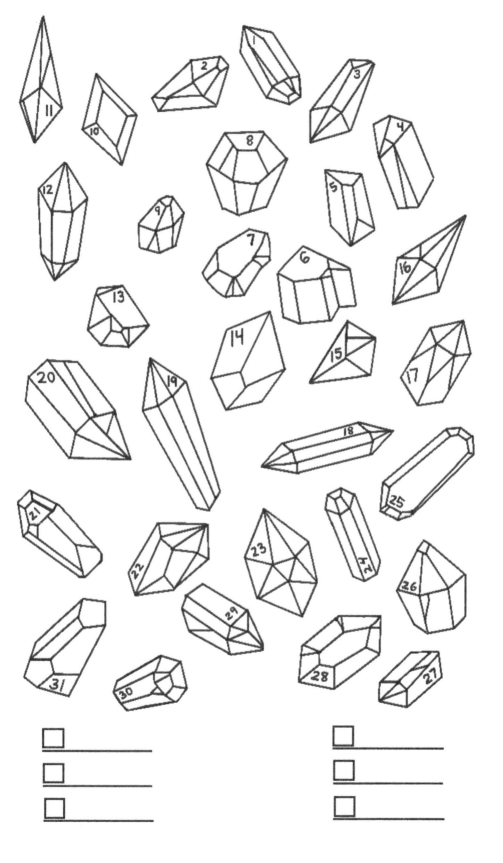

Month: **Year:**

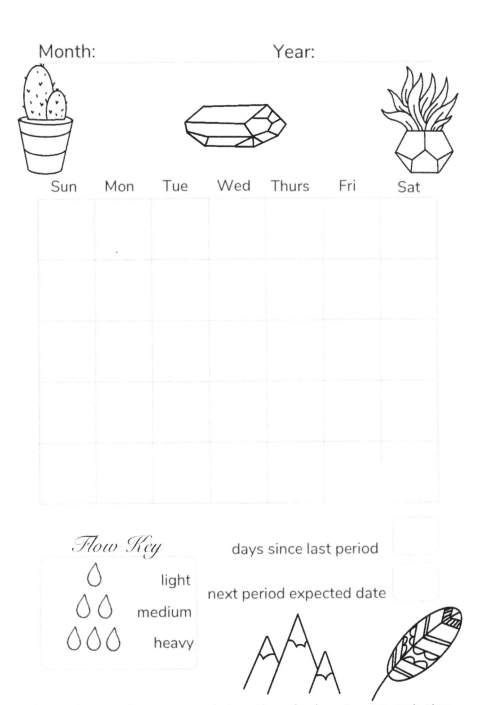

Sun	Mon	Tue	Wed	Thurs	Fri	Sat

Flow Key

light

medium

heavy

days since last period

next period expected date

Mark the days you have your period on the calendar. You can mark them
using the flow key or draw hearts, stars or anything you like.

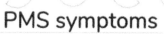

PMS symptoms

Write down anything you may be experiencing during your period. Include your moods, any cravings, aches, cramps or tenderness you are feeling and anything you did that helped.

Day 1	
Day 2	
Day 3	
Day 4	
Day 5	
Day 6	
Day 7	

Notes:

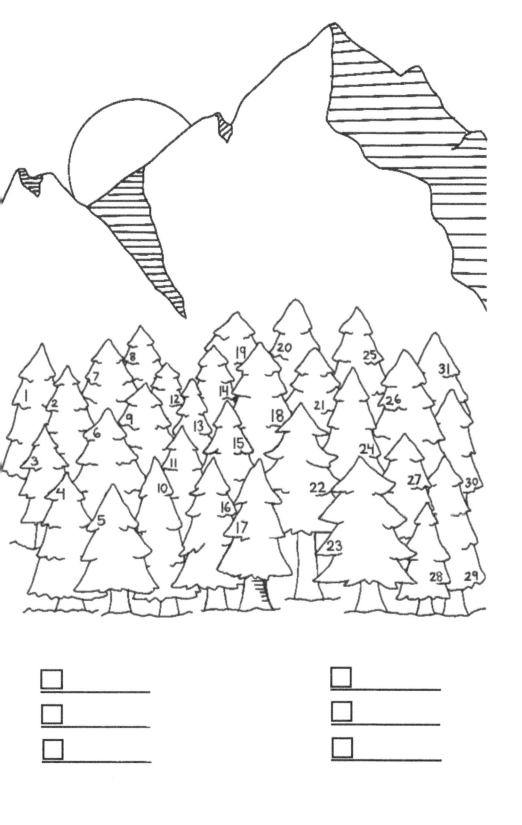

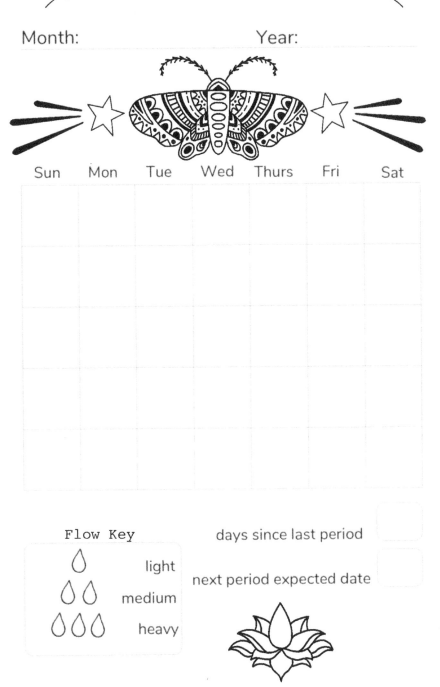

Month: _____   **Year:** _____

Sun	Mon	Tue	Wed	Thurs	Fri	Sat

Flow Key

◊ light

◊◊ medium

◊◊◊ heavy

_____ days since last period

_____ next period expected date

Mark the days you have your period on the calendar. You can mark them using the flow key or draw hearts, stars or anything you like.

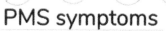

PMS symptoms

Write down anything you may be experiencing during your period. Include your moods, any cravings, aches, cramps or tenderness you are feeling and anything you did that helped.

Day 1	
Day 2	
Day 3	
Day 4	
Day 5	
Day 6	
Day 7	

Notes:

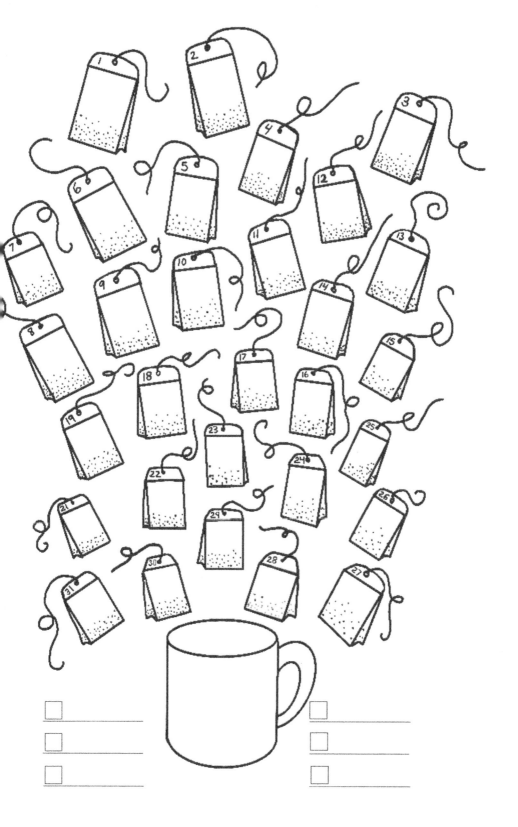

Month: _____   Year: _____

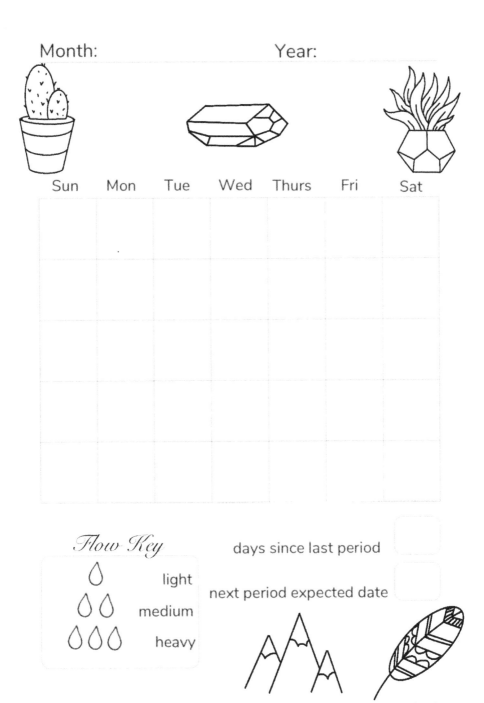

Sun	Mon	Tue	Wed	Thurs	Fri	Sat

Flow Key

◊ light

◊ ◊ medium

◊ ◊ ◊ heavy

days since last period [ ]

next period expected date [ ]

Mark the days you have your period on the calendar. You can mark them using the flow key or draw hearts, stars or anything you like.

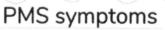

PMS symptoms

Write down anything you may be experiencing during your period. Include your moods, any cravings, aches, cramps or tenderness you are feeling and anything you did that helped.

Day 1	
Day 2	
Day 3	
Day 4	
Day 5	
Day 6	
Day 7	

Notes:

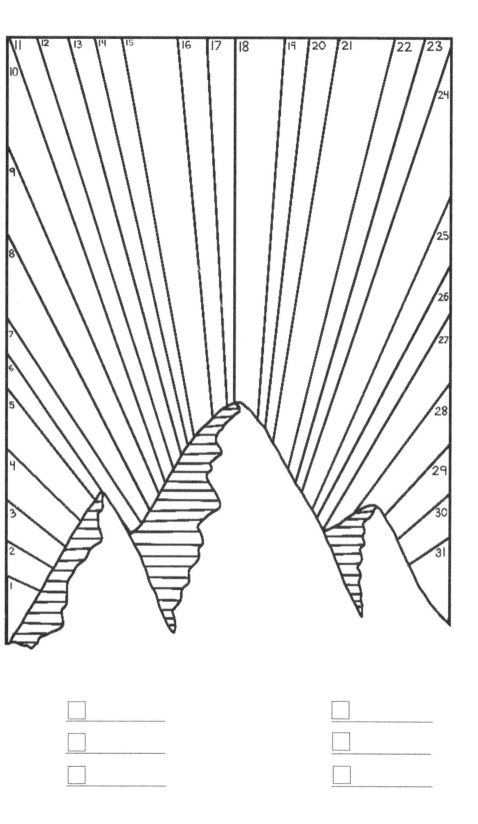

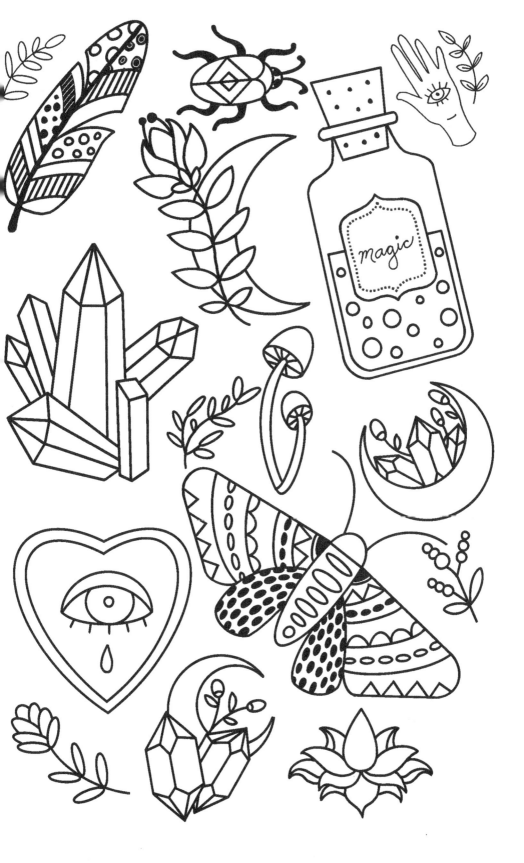

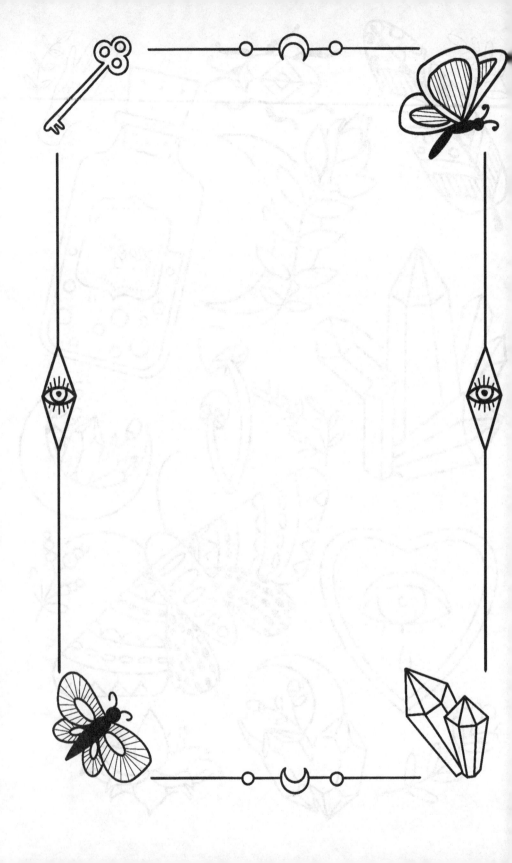

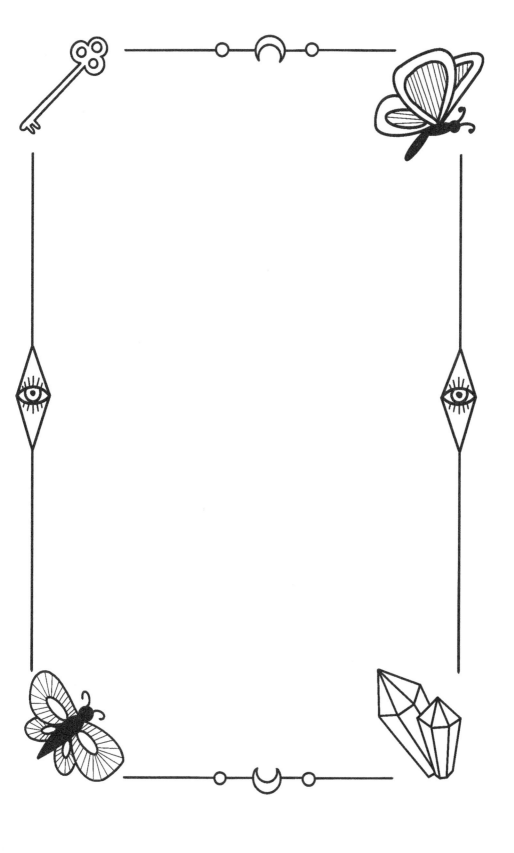

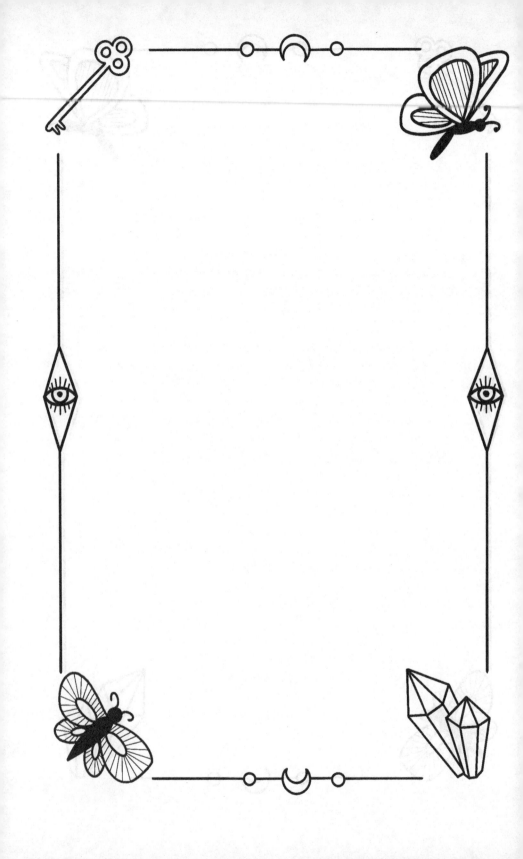

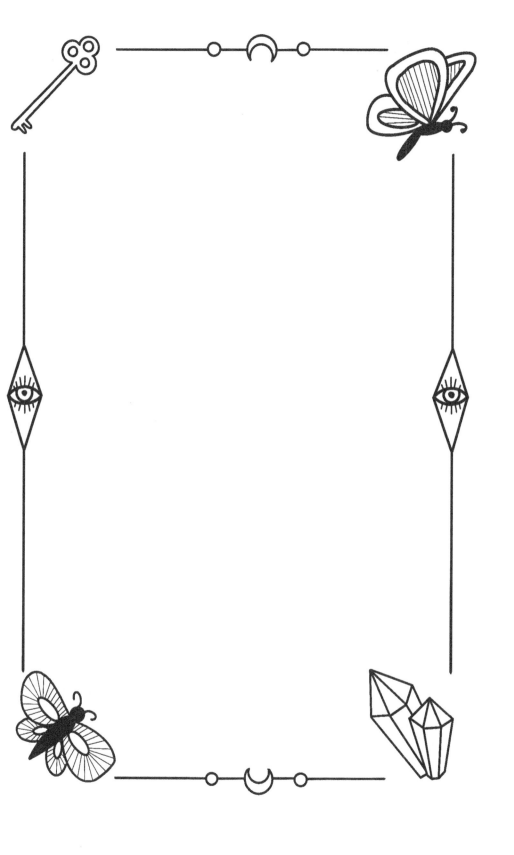

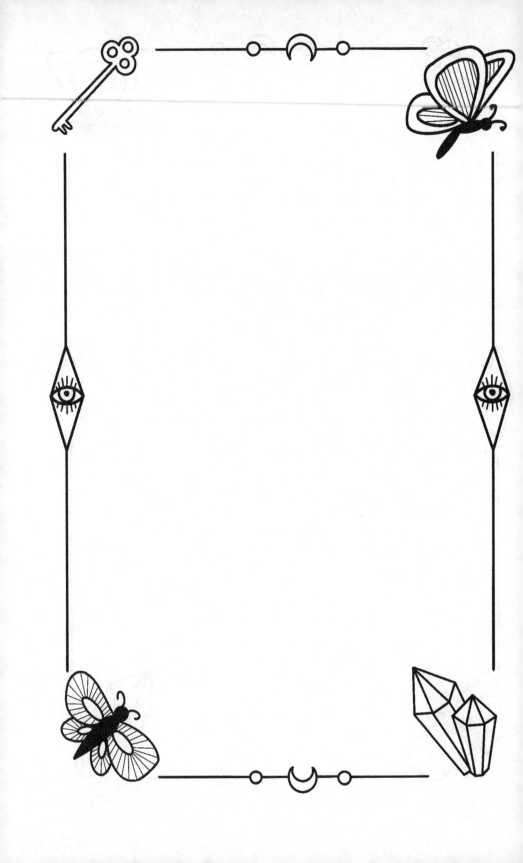

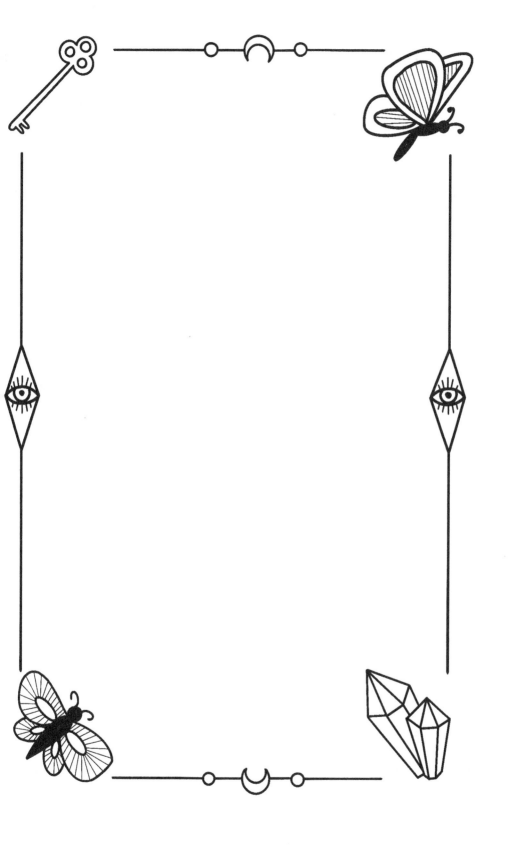

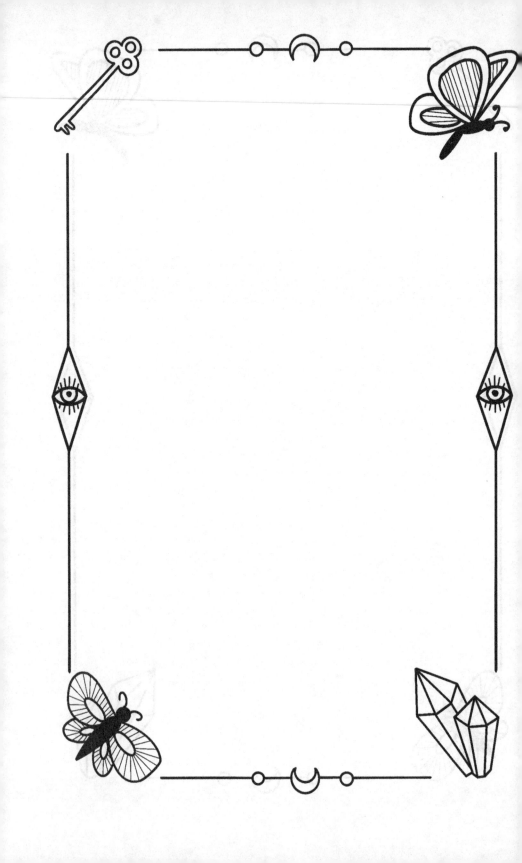

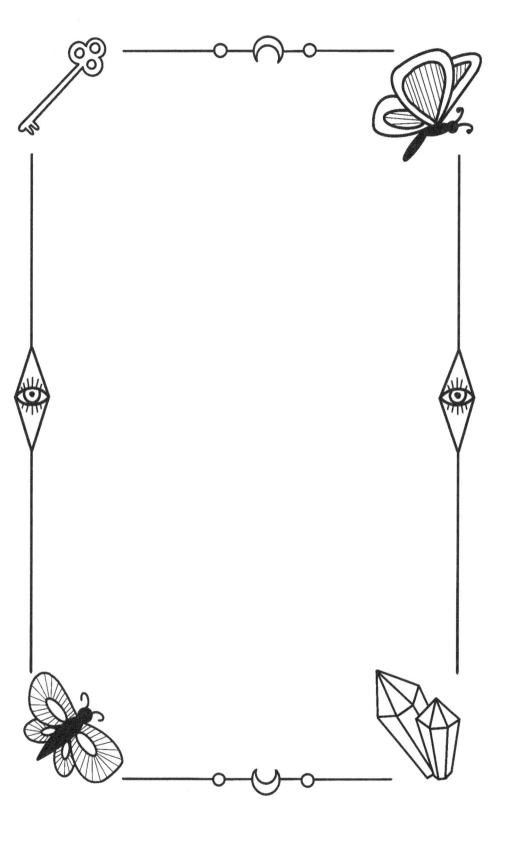

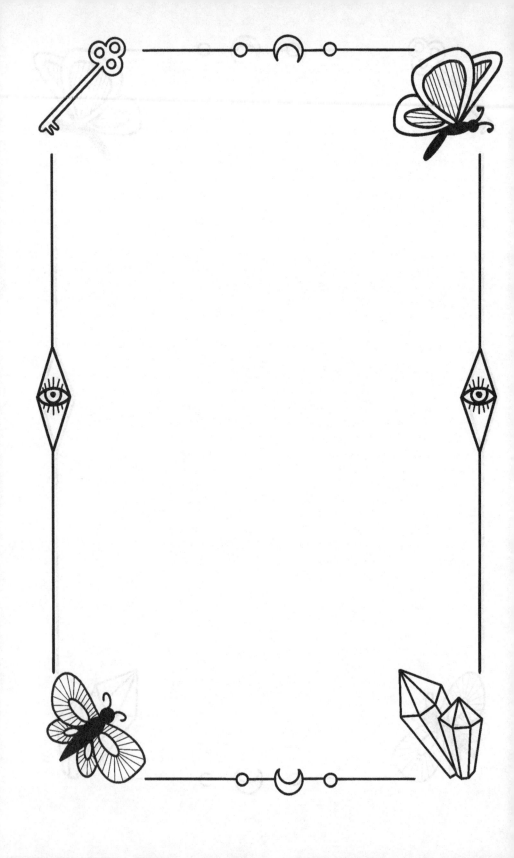

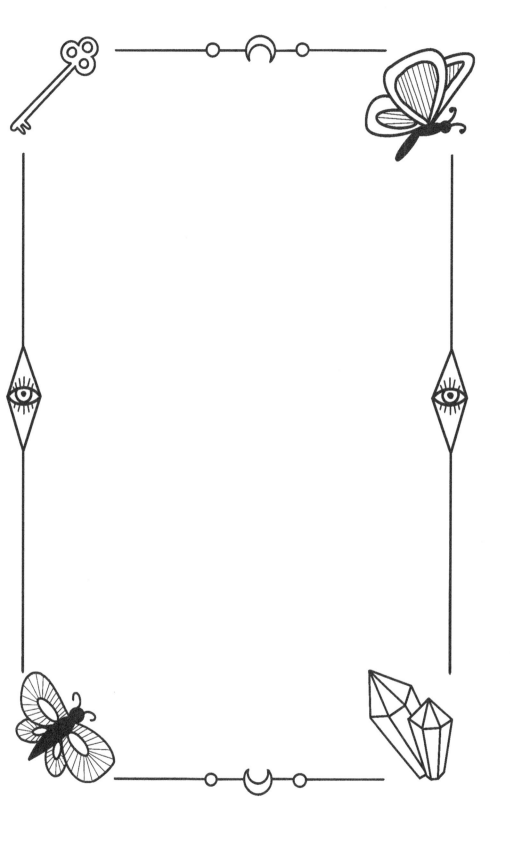

Made in the USA
Monee, IL
17 November 2024

70353768R00056